Creating Compassion

A 7 Week Guide to Build a Healthier, Happier, & More Peaceful You

Through

the 7 Mirrors of Compassion

Alexander Puhalla Ph.D.
&
Cyril Puhalla M.D.

Made in United States
Copyright © 2024
Cyril Puhalla MD
Alexander Puhalla PhD
All rights reserved.
ISBN: 9798339064374
Imprint: Independently published

Dedication

To our parents and grandparents for teaching us the basics to survive, be healthy, happy & help all others

ACKNOWLEDGMENTS

Acknowledging all our teachers who taught us all they could, our students who taught us more & our patients who taught us the most & what the others could not

A special acknowledgement to Dr. Jean Arlt, Dr. Alex's wife & Dr. Cyril's daughter-in-law, as she provided vital feedback during the creation and editing of this book.

Compassion is engaging in presence with the Connected Self

> Our minds naturally want to push away the necessary suffering of life through rejecting what we do not like, distracting ourselves with what brings temporary happiness, and ignoring what is not immediately satisfying. Through mindful practice we can learn to catch ourselves when these automatic cycles occur to remove the unnecessary suffering that this avoidance brings. Through this self-growth, which is the only thing we have control over, we can learn to engage with the connected versus separate self by activating our natural humane instincts of compassion, kindness, and altruism. Through this we can learn to be happy, healthy, and more peaceful.

Table of Contents

7 WEEKS TO A HAPPIER, HEALTHIER, & PEACEFUL YOU 1

NECESSARY VS. UNNECESSARY SUFFERING: THE BASICS 3
    SUMMARY OF "THE 12 LAWS" (PUHALLA & PUHALLA, 2023) 6

CONNECTED SELF: NO AVOIDANCE ALLOWED 9

1. LEARNING TO LIVE IN THE MOMENT 15
    STEPS TO CALM MEDITATIVE BREATHING 18
    STEPS TO CALMING IMAGERY 19
        Alternative Mindfulness Training Activities 21

2. ACCEPTANCE IS THE WAY 25
    NAIL A BET: A Mindful Tool for Emotional Healing 26
    STEPS TO ACCEPTANCE BASED IMAGERY 32

3. HOLDING ON TO THE PAST ONLY DRAINS 35
    LET IT COME, LET IT BE, LET IT GO MEDITATION 37
    STEPS TO LETTING GO BASED IMAGERY 38

4. SELF-LOVE FOR SELF-GROWTH 41
    LOVING KINDNESS MEDITATION 45
    STEPS TO LOVING KINDNESS IMAGERY 48

5. CREATE THE JOY YOU SEEK 51
    MEDITATION ON RADICAL ACCEPTANCE: 55
    RADICAL ACCEPTANCE IMAGERY EXERCISE: 56

6. UNIFICATION VERSUS SEPARATION 59
    QUESTIONS TO CONTEMPLATE FOR UNIFYING WHOLESOME CHOICES 62
    STEPS TO UNIFICATION IMAGERY 66

7. COMPASSION BEYOND EMPATHY 69
    COMPASSIONATE SELF EXERCISES 73
    STEPS TO PERFECT NURTURER IMAGERY (LEE, 2005) 76

RESOURCES AND RECOMMENDED READINGS 81

APPENDIX 83

7 Weeks to a Happier, Healthier, and More Peaceful You

This book has a dual purpose. The primary being to help anyone who would like to live a happier and more connected life through accessing the compassionate self. This will be done by integrating mindfulness based and compassion focused techniques that will be suggested for a week at a time. As such, each chapter can be read at the beginning of the week to introduce a new set of concepts that will build on each other, as well as exercises that will help strengthen one's compassion muscle. Of course, if you need longer than a week to refine a specific set of skills that is perfectly fine, however, these mindfulness based and compassion focused techniques are skills that one will need to practice across one's life so that they can be automatic in nature. In this, an individual can use this book to learn to accept the dissatisfaction that may be present in *"the way it is"* versus *"the way they want it to be"* and find greater compassion, connection and kindness within themselves and others. Through this, one can learn to dissolve the negative *"self-talk"* or deep seeded shame that may be holding them back from a healthier, happier, and more peaceful life.

"The Compassionate Connected Self finds peace in the certainty of the here and now, versus the Separate Self looking to past experiences or an uncertain, fantasized future."

The second purpose of this book is to provide a basic framework of engaging in Compassion Focused interventions in an individual or group structure. Compassion based techniques (e.g., Au et al., 2017) and Compassion Focused Therapy (CFT; Gilbert, 2009) both are found to help reduce anxiety, depression, and posttraumatic stress disorder (PTSD) symptoms, as well as a plethora of other conditions (Millard et al., 2023). Specifically, compassion techniques appear to be especially strong against shame (i.e., an emotion connected to negative thoughts about oneself).

This book's unique angle is utilizing the seven mirrors of compassion, which are based on Buddhist mindfulness-based principles (e.g., Hochswender, Martin, & Morino, 2001), to build a basic structure.

This book will increase (a) cognitive awareness of necessary versus unnecessary suffering, (b) cognitive control / acceptance through sitting with and letting go of not only negative emotional experiences, but of equal importance, those judged as positive, and (c) cognitive-affective flexibility and regulation through learning to dissolve negative emotions using compassion, kindness, and acts of altruism. However, the first goal is learning the process within oneself before applying it to others. Thus, it is strongly suggested to build one's own self-compassion practice first.

> *"The energy we put into the world will return in like manner, however, only in its own time."*

With these dual purposes in mind the book will have a simple structure:

1. <u>Intellectual learning:</u> A new concept or mirror will be introduced with some basic philosophy of why it is important to one's health, happiness, and sense of peace.
2. <u>Applied learning:</u> A technique will be provided to practice the core of the concept / mirror.
3. <u>Experiential learning:</u> A meditative training will be provided that can be conducted daily to assist with this process.

The question you may all be asking is:

> *"Well, how much of this do I have to do to feel better?"*

The answer is different for each person, but the more we keep asking that question instead of attempting to engage in self-growth, the longer it will be. Practice these therapeutic techniques and meditations once per day for a minimum of 5 minutes, and over time it will build from a singular moment of relief to a skill, and from a skill to an automatic response, and from an automatic response to a way of life.

> *"Building compassion and altruism for oneself and others is no different than building any other muscle, it just takes consistency, patience, and repeated practice."*

Necessary vs. Unnecessary Suffering: The Basics

The purpose of this book is to focus on the Mirror of Dharma (Gyatso, 2018). Dharma basically means *"the way it is"* as it is happening in the here and now. It is related to broader Buddhist philosophy with the goal to build compassion. Multiple practices have broken down this mirror into seven, which we will do as well. However, to properly utilize these mirrors for the purpose of building compassion to dissolve one's darker emotions and thoughts, one must have a basic understanding of Buddhist philosophy.

Several books have been recommended in the reference section, as well as a previous book on this topic by the authors (Puhalla & Puhalla, 2023). What follows is an abbreviated version of the first chapter of that book that provides a broad overview of how we end up adding unnecessary suffering to our lives by attempting to avoid the necessary suffering. This may be more than enough for the average reader, however, please refer to this section as needed.

Helpful natural suffering is a normal reaction to emotional and physical pain. The full mindful experience of this suffering is not an option.

However, because we don't fully experience this helpful suffering, we can end up creating harmful suffering that adds more pain and suffering in a cyclical fashion. For example, we all have moments where we empathize with a sick loved one or have concern for them, however, we add suffering when we attempt to avoid it through rejecting the associated painful emotions representing *"the way it is"* and simultaneously distracting ourselves with more positive things (e.g., in the form of alcohol, media, food, & etc.).

Through this, we end up with a positive feedback loop that adds more suffering as feelings of depression, anxiety, and shame. We all do this temporarily, however, when we keep encouraging the cycle versus accepting the reality as it is by activating the compassionate connected self, the suffering can reach harmful levels.

One way to prevent or remove this harmful unnecessary suffering is through accepting the reality as it is versus the way one wants it to be and activating the compassionate self. To do this, we must learn to become compassionate on three levels:

1) Intellectually (i.e., through thoughts)

2) Applied (i.e., through behaviour)

3) Experienced (i.e., while mindful)

While not fully covered in this book, below is a figure of the 12 basic laws of the mind so that as you practice your mindfulness, and compassion exercises you will have greater understanding of cause and effect. Use this figure as a reference to return to as needed, for it is the basis on which the Mirrors are derived using information from all the Laws being Connected and working together. The 7 Mirrors are not only an expansion of Law 5 but of all 12 Laws. The Laws can be looked at as if they provide a general strategy to life, while the 7 Mirrors give one specific tactics to deal with pains and suffering of living.

Figure 1. The 12 Basic Laws

The Laws represent "the way it is," though 12 separate principles that are interconnected.

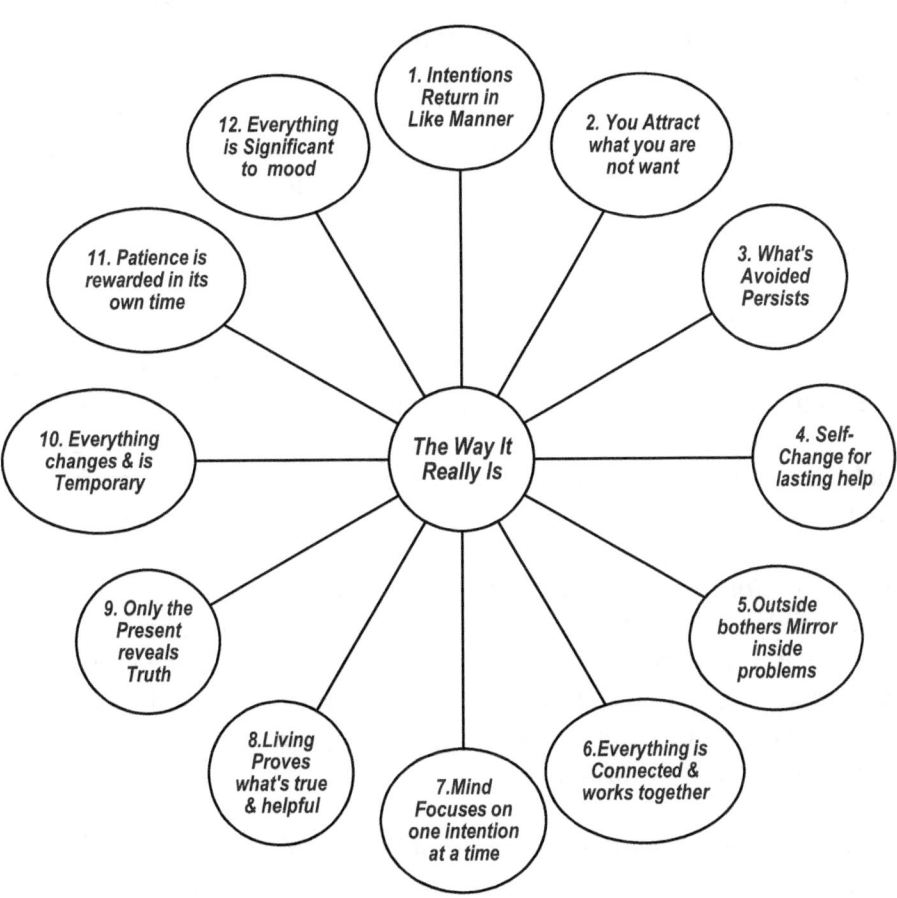

Summary of "The 12 Laws" (Puhalla & Puhalla, 2023)

According to many philosophical perspectives (e.g., radical determinism, Buddhist philosophy, Hinduism), the reality we live in is self-determined or created based on our internal and external experiences of the world. As such, we develop biases and beliefs on how we want it to be versus the way it really is. These laws allow us to break the chain and begin accepting reality as it is, while the mirrors will provide active skills and techniques to dissolve or combat the toxic energy, that has developed in response to the cycle of avoidance, that leads to unnecessary suffering. Below are brief definitions (note: please see Puhalla & Puhalla, 2023 for more details)

Law 1 - Intentions always return in like manner
Simply, do no purposeful harm, as the energy of intentions you send into the world matter and always return to you. In other words, even the smallest intention or response may have returning effects. When we generally send out helpful and loving intentions, helpful and loving intentions will return in their own time. However, if we send out hateful and angry intentions, then that is what will be returned in their own time.

Law 2 - Mind attracts what you are, not what you want
The Mind will attract all energy, positive negative or neutral, whether you want it to or not. For example, if you make the choice to be kind, that energy will be stored in your mind to attract more kindness. If you have intentions of violence or anger, its energy will be attracted to you whether you want it or not.

Law 3 - What is avoided or resisted will persist
Even when we believe that we have avoided or pushed away a negative emotion or thought, it is still there. In fact, sooner or later it will come back and (often) at a greater intensity. Thus, whatever you resist will persist.

Law 4 - Self-change as a priority for help that lasts
If you change what is in your mind, then you will not have to change your body, others, or the outside world. If others are violent to you, it is easier to remove the violent energy in yourself than in them.

Law 5 - Life's bothers mirrors what is already in your mind
Generally, what bothers you the most in the outside world is what you need to focus on internally first.

Law 6 - Everything is connected and works together
Everything, without exception, is connected. Our mind's energy is connected to the body, which is connected to our actions, which is connected to all others, the outside world and all we do in the outside world.

Law 7 - Mind can have one single focus on one intention at a time
Our body must multitask to survive, however, the more our mind is "split" keep the parts separate from the whole, the more cyclic unnecessary suffering we endure. You cannot have the intention to be helpful & harmful, or to love & hate in the same mind moment. As such, if you apply mindfulness to focus on peaceful, compassionate, and altruistic intentions, then overtime this can act as a neutralizer for harmful intentions.

Law 8 – Life will prove beliefs either false or true
Over time our choices will provide evidence for or against our beliefs. While overly simple, sooner or later the intentions and energy we put into the world will provide internal and external evidence of them being helpful or harmful.

Law 9 - Only in the present is the truth of happiness revealed
The only moment is the present moment, with both memories of the past and thoughts of the future occurring in the here and now. Thus, happiness can only be found in the present, because it is an experience of the present, which is why the goal is to engage in compassionate and connected ways with oneself and others to continue this energy forward.

Law 10 - Everything is temporary and changing
Every experience, neutral, positive, or negative, arises into awareness, occurs, and moves on to end. No moment will be identical in nature and the more we live in the present moment, the more joy and happiness we can find.

Law 11- Patience is always rewarded in its own time
Patience is required to reap the benefits of compassion and altruism, as evidence for one's positive intentions will only come in its own time. Additionally, patience with practice is the best pathway towards self-growth and the most powerful antidote for the most destructive emotion, anger.

Law 12 - Everything, no matter how small, is significant to the mood
All intentions matter, no matter how small or large. The way you practice or engage in one moment, over time, is how we engage with them all.

Connected Self: No Avoidance Allowed

Avoidance through <u>rejecting</u> of what we do not like (e.g., shame, guilt, anger, unwanted memories), over <u>indulging</u> in what we like too much (e.g., over indulging with foods, drugs, sex, and media), and <u>ignoring</u> what seems mundane or boring (e.g., scrolling through social media while on an elevator) is unknowingly increasing uncessary suffering for us, others, and those we care about in our lives. As such, avoidance of the *"the way it is"* becomes automatically harmful when the intentions are selfish and lead us to being separate from others, while accepting it and applying the seven mirrors can lead to greater feelings of connectedness and happiness (i.e., connected self).

The goal of this book is to learn to disolve the darkness within, but before we can do that we must understand, once again, that we can only have a single intention at time, which means we can either prioritize holding on to suffering, through avoiding the initial pain, or make it a priority for the mind to accept it, allow it to be as it is, so through experience we can let go of suffering to focus on compassion, kindess, sharing, and acceptance. In other words, if you are attempting to learn these techinques with any mixed motivations, you may still be sending negative intentions into the world! However, if you are doing this for the purpose of growth, then you are already on the right path and beginning to intellectually understand.

Below is a partial list comparing the Separate Self & the Connected Self based on their effects as Harmful or Helpful. Come back to review this figure frequently, for it summarizes most of what you need to know about the Separate Self and its cycle of Self-Desrtuctiveness that leads to illlness, suffering and premature death, and the energy of the Connected Self of Compassion and its path of Wellbeing leading to higher levels of health, happiness, and a peaceful mind.

If one understands and follows the 12 Laws of the mind and applies the 7 Mirrors of Compassion, one is on the path of wellness, but even if one law or mirror is not followed, the result is that of cycles of Self-Destructiveness.

Figure 2. Removing harm of Cyclic Self-Destructiveness by Letting Go of Attachments of Separate Self with Compassion

Cycle of Self-Destructiveness: Separate Self	Steps for Health, Happiness, & Peace: Connected Self
☐ Unaware that avoiding painful feelings of *"the way it is"* is harmful	☐ Mindful awareness of harm of avoidance
☐ Pain is not *"what I want"*	☐ Pains accepted mindfully with compassion
☐ Only perceive what I want as the pleasures & avoid pains	☐ *"the way it really is"* there is no pleasure without pain, no pain without pleasure
☐ Separate oneself from pains	☐ Stay connected to pain & pleasure
☐ Desire makes new pleasure exist & pain not exist over humane values	☐ Humane intentions towards kindness, sharing, and connection
☐ Become trapped in thinking mode to avoid the reality as it is.	☐ Shift from thinking to mindful dissolving & compassion
☐ New feelings personalized as friend or foe	☐ Feelings as impersonal energy
☐ Attach to new feelings to ignore neutrals	☐ Let feelings fully come
☐ Over indulge in positves & reject negatives	☐ Let feelings be as they are
☐ Seperate self becomes more powerful	☐ Compassion feeling of painful energy to let the attachment go!
☐ Life's solutions contaminated with uncertainty, fear, depression, addiction & anger	☐ No extra uncertainty, fear, depression, addictivness, & anger
☐ Self is unaware of harmful avoidance which fuels a new cycle	☐ No Cycle - instead Health, Happiness, & Peace Of Mind

Exercise for the Week: Notice One's Emotions & Reactions

What do I mean by emotions?
By emotions I mean the physical reaction that occurs in response to internal and external stimuli, which include various systems. Generally, emotions can be described in one word and can either be positive or negative, strong or faint, and usually have thoughts and behavioral urges connected to them, but are not the emotion itself. For example, anxiety generally is connected to increased heart rate, sweating, rapid / irregular resipriation, and difficulty focusing (i.e., urge to flee). Compartively, anger is often related to increased heart rate, physical tension, and (at times) being overly focused in on what one is angry about (i.e., urge to fight). Some emotions occur after we begin to interpret a situation as well (e.g., shame, guilt, & pride).

NAIL Those Emotions:
Before we can even remove the unnecessary suffering one may just want to begin to notice emotional reactions and responses to them. As such, over the next week the goal is:

1. <u>Notice</u> in the <u>Now</u> what emotion you are experiencing.
2. <u>Accept & Allow</u> it to occur without attempting to avoid it.
3. <u>Investigate</u> the thoughts / behavioral urges experienced.
4. <u>Learn</u> how your emotional reactions may trigger specific thoughts and behavioral urges and how that may determine how you interact with yourself, others, and the world.

Example:

1. Notice: the anger when someone cuts you off in traffic.
2. Allow: Just notice the emotional state (no immediate reaction).
3. Investigate: It bothers you as it is unfair and they are rude, per your preception.
4. Learn: Your natural reaction is to act aggressively, however, by just providing some time from the emotion, that desire weakens. Later you may learn to use compassion to also dissolve this state (e.g., What are other compassionate reasons they may have cut you off?).

Exercise for the Week: Notice Now to Begin to Grow
Complete this NAIL assignment once per day to become more aware, accepting, and allowing of emotions (see figure 3).

Figure 3. Emotion Log (NAIL made simple):

Date	**N**otice & Allow (Emotion)	**I**nvestigate (Thoughts / Urges)	**L**earn (Usual reaction vs. Alternatives)
8/10/24	Anxiety Fear	I am going to fail this test no matter what. Avoid studying	Usually I will focus on my anxiety or do something else. I could just sit and study for a bit.

1. Learning to Live in the Moment

Breath, Breath, Distract & Repeat…

"Presence is the ability to just be with "the way it is" without judgement."

Mirror 1 - Reflects the Truth of a Mindful Perpetual Present

Our problems occur over and over because we hold on to the pain of our Body sensations, Emotions, & Thoughts (BETs) that end up being stored in our mind and body, which eventually fuel the same cycle later. During this process we attempt to avoid the necessary suffering of life, which overtime adds harmful suffering. Comparatively, if we allow the negative energy to naturally end then we would not add suffering and thereby begin to live a more peaceful life.

For example, conditions arise that may make you feel anxious about telling a friend or partner that something they do hurts your feelings. At first you contemplate approaching them about this, however, you begin to add unnecessary harmful mental energy as you worry about their past reactions to arguments and projecting towards the future of how they might react. Eventually you either (a) work yourself up into a state that may increase the probability of an argument or (b) avoid the discussion all together. This then will make you much more likely to continue with the same pattern in the future instead of being honest with yourself and your loved one. Thus, rejecting the reality *"as it is,"* with its unpleasant emotions that you have been conditioned to automatically avoid.

This happens because you are not being responsive to the present but are being distracted by past experiences and future wants. If your mind was trained to stay mindfully present, you would still remember and learn from your previous experience but not react to it automatically.

Automatic Reactions to the Past versus Present Responsiveness
One way to begin becoming more peaceful in the here and now, as well as compassionate towards yourself and others, is to modify this automatic reaction to the past by staying aware of your feelings in each present moment. One way to practice this is through mindful breathing and learning to be present with each component of the breath.

Remember, a mirror doesn't reflect the past and has no expectations for anything in the future. Its reflections exists only in the perpetual present. Your mind in its "true nature" is like a mirror that would reflect only what is happening. Instead we are conditioned for the mind to be more like a sponge, that holds on, and we allow things to soak in. Of course, there are similarities of past moments to the present (e.g., we all have had many difficult conversations with loved ones), however, there are always differences that must be noticed and fully taken in. Thus, before we can become compassionate and kind, we must fully consider what enters the mind (a.k.a. mind-full-ness) in the present moment. Let emotion fully come, then let it just be as it is, experience its energy fully, so it is all used up, then you can let it go!

The Mirrors of Compassion summarize seven qualities of mindful perpetual presence in life, accepting, letting go, selflessness, creativity, unifying, and compassion. The goal is to practice these qualities within both our mindful meditative practice and daily living to remove unnecessary suffering.

"We can learn from the past but choose not to have our beliefs frozen in time. Always modify the present truth with the intention to be wholesomely helpful towards our connected self and others."

Exercise for the Week #1: Breath, Breath, Distract, & Repeat

Meditative Exercise for Mirror #1

The goal this week is to begin adding at least <u>15 minutes a day of meditative practice.</u> The practice can be broken into 5 minute periods, or even less. For some even practicing 1 minute each hour can be helpful. Even one breath mindfully experienced is helpful and a good start. Just like a child walks one step at a time, you take one breath at a time. Of course, more may lead to greater benefits, however, 15-20 minutes per day is usually enough to begin to notice the calming effects of meditation. As the breath is with us constantly, it is a terrific anchor in the here and now. However, even the greatest meditators will become distracted and so will you! The goal is not to stay focused just on the breath, but to accept with a sense of forgiveness that you will become distracted and gently return the breath.

If I ever become upset with this process or begin to judge it or myself, I often ask how would I respond to a loved one who says they are *"too anxious to try this"* or *"I am just not strong enough to do it,"* or think *"I just can't stay focused on the exercise, it is too hard... boring... relaxing"* and treat myself how I would treat them. Below are the ABC-Ds of meditative breathing. Remember just breath, breath, and (when distracted) repeat.

Concentrative Mediation using Breathing is as simple as ABC:
1. Become **A**ware of your **B**reathing. Make your breath your only focus as you feel it mindfully. Mindfully means stay in the present with no thinking, which takes you automatically to the past and future.
2. Doing this develops **C**oncentration with calmness and alertness.
3. This concentration will be broken with a **D**istraction by thinking. Just simply acknowledge the distraction, you may want to label it by saying to yourself "thinking, thinking" regardless if it is positive, negative, or neutral, and return to the physical sensation of the breath.

Meditation has unique properties that cannot be duplicated by any drug.

"Calming drugs make you less alert, alerting ones make you tense, only meditation will lead to being both alert and calm."

Steps to Calm Meditative Breathing

Center yourself by taking several deep breaths, potentially counting each one as you get in comfortable position.

1. Slowly take a deep breath in to pull yourself into the present moment.
2. Hold it for a second and feel the alert tension.
3. Let the breath slowly go and feel the sense of calm.
4. Stay **A**ware of each **B**reath as it is happening without thought, judgement, or behavioral reaction.
5. Only **C**oncentrate on feeling the breath with no thinking.
6. Repeat the ***ABCs*** over & over, for as long as you need.
7. You will become **D**istracted by something:
   a. Positives
      i. Examples: thoughts about a meal, seeing a friend, or something you are excited about; A sensation of a cool breeze coming over you or even the relaxing sensation of the deep breathing.
   b. Negatives
      i. Examples: a thought about the exercise being boring, or you're doing it wrong. Memories from the past that you feel guilt, shame, or sadness over. Worries or dread about the future. Physical aches, pains, or itches.
   c. Neutrals
      i. Boredom over the alert calming state you are in.
8. Accept the distraction as *"the way it is"* and return to feel the breath.
9. Simply breathe, breathe, become distracted, and repeat over and over.

Steps to Calming Imagery

Similar to the deep breathing exercise, individuals who have strong visualization may benefit from using guided or self-guided imagery. Below are basic instructions on how to attempt guided imagery based on the same principles. Apply these steps after a few minutes of deep breathing.

1. Slowly begin to visualize a calm lake. The lake can be real, or it can be an item of your imagination. In this exercise, B of the ABC's stands for anything you can single focus on, like the lake.

2. Visualize the calmness of the water, by providing visual details of what you see. You may also visualize the scenery around the lake if it helps you become centered.

3. As you observe the lake continue to slowly breath in and out.

4. Imagine the lake is the current state of your mind with the calmness representing engaging in presence (i.e., being only in the here and now).

5. Become **A**ware of the calmness of the lake and only **C**oncentrate on the visualization of the lake, with your breath as an anchor.

6. What do you see on the lake? Around the lake? What does the calmness of the lake look like?

7. Breathe in, and out as your only focus is on the lake's calmness.

8. You will become **D**istracted by something:
    a. Positives
        i. Examples: other beautiful or notable pictures in your imagery. Beliefs of how well you are doing or something happening in the future. Feelings of relaxation.
    b. Negatives

      i. Examples: thoughts that you are doing the exercise wrong. Memories of the past. Worries or fears about the future. Beliefs that you will never get this or learn to dissolve the darkness within or other negative thoughts about yourself. Traumas from your past, or the negative emotionality around the trauma / memory.

   c. Neutral
      i. Boredom over this or anything else. Physical stimuli that pulls you out the exercise.

9. Visualize these distractions as tiny ripples in the lake, with larger or stronger distractions as bigger ripples or even waves.

10. Allow them to naturally occur without judgement. Return to the peaceful state of the lake in your mind's eye. Repeat this process.

11. As you repeat this process you will become distracted again, and you may even need to pause for a second and call out the distraction.

12. Gently return to the exercise, utilizing your breath or the instructions as an anchor of the here and now.

13. **Repeat** for about 15-20 minutes.

Either exercise can count as part of your weekly meditative practice. However, the goal of learning to become calm during meditation is also to find this state in day-to-day life. Attempt to find an **additional** 15 minutes where you are present in the here and now during other activities. These can include mindful conversations with loved ones, mindful eating, mindful engagement in exercise, or even mindful engagement in hobbies (e.g., woodworking, biking, fishing, swimming, writing, & etc..). Below are some examples of other mindfulness activities one can do with brief instructions. Please use figure 4 to assist with this process.

Alternative Mindfulness Training Activities

1. **Mindful Walking**

    o **Steps to Remove Harmful Feelings:**

    1. Choose a quiet, safe place to walk, either indoors or outdoors.

    2. Begin walking slowly, paying attention to each step. Notice how your feet feel as they make contact with the ground.

    3. As you walk, allow your mind to focus on the sensation of movement rather than any troubling thoughts.

    4. If thoughts related to guilt or shame arise, acknowledge them, then gently return your focus to your steps.

    5. Walk mindfully for 10-15 minutes, allowing your body and mind to work together in releasing emotions.

    o **Steps to Build Compassionate States:**

    1. While walking, reflect on a positive quality you wish to cultivate, such as kindness or forgiveness.

    2. With each step, imagine walking towards this quality, embodying it with your movements.

    3. As you walk, mentally repeat phrases like *"May I be kind"* or *"May I forgive"* to reinforce these states.

    4. Walk with intention for 10-15 minutes, nurturing these helpful qualities.

2. **Mindful Journaling**
    - **Steps to Remove Harmful Feelings:**
        1. Set aside 10-15 minutes in a quiet space where you won't be disturbed.
        2. Begin by writing down any thoughts or feelings that are troubling you. Allow your words to flow without censorship.
        3. Once you've expressed your feelings, review what you've written. Notice any patterns or recurring themes.
        4. Reflect on how these thoughts might be influencing your emotions and behavior.
        5. Conclude by writing a few sentences about how you can let go of these harmful emotions, using a compassionate tone towards yourself.
    - **Steps to Build Compassionate States:**
        1. After journaling about harmful feelings, shift your focus to writing about positive qualities you want to develop, like compassion or forgiveness.
        2. Write about times when you've experienced these feelings, either towards yourself or others.
        3. Reflect on how you can cultivate these qualities more in your daily life.
        4. End your journaling session by writing an affirmation or intention for the day, such as "Today, I choose kindness."

3. **Mindful Eating**

    o **Steps to Remove Harmful Feelings:**

    1. Choose a meal or snack to eat mindfully, without distractions like TV or smartphones.

    2. Before eating, take a moment to appreciate the food in front of you, noticing its colors, textures, and aromas.

    3. Experience each sense without judgement.

    4. As you eat, chew slowly and pay attention to the taste and sensation of each bite.

    5. If judgements about what you are eating, or other things, arise, gently let them come, be, and go.

    6. Use this time to ground yourself in the present moment, reducing the influence of negative feelings.

    o **Steps to Build Compassionate States:**

    1. Begin your mindful eating practice by setting an intention, such as "*I nourish my body with kindness.*"

    2. With each bite, focus on how the food is providing your body with energy and health.

    3. Express gratitude for the meal, considering all the people and processes involved in bringing it to your table.

    4. Allow the experience of mindful eating to reinforce feelings of compassion towards yourself and others.

Figure 4. Mindfulness Practice Log

Date	Meditation Practice	Mindful Living Practice	Notes (how did engaging in presence feel or effect you?)
8/17/24	3x today for 5 minutes. 1x at bedtime.	While swimming I only paid attention to my body's experience	1. It helped me fall alseep. 2. When I did it before my meeting I was calmer. 3. I enjoyed my breakfast more.

2. Acceptance is the Way

Accept the soil as it is, so we can learn to sow

Accept "the way it is" versus what the separate self "wants it to be."

Mirror 2 - A Mirror Accepts All Things Without Judgement

A mirror simply accepts the reality *"as it is"* instead of judging what it reflects. It does not choose to reflect off emotional biases based on past positive, negative, or neutral experiences. It accepts all equally. When we engage in kindness towards ourselves and others, as our Connected Compassionate Self, through non-judgmental acceptance it relieves the weighty burden of unnecessary suffering.

The primary issue is when we are faced with moments that we disagree with, we attempt to avoid through rejection of negatives, overindulgence of positives, and ignoring the neutral. This avoidance allows us to shift the reality *"as it is"* to a more selfish perception of the *"way we want it to be."* For example, we all have moments when we feel disliked by others and even rejected. Think of harsh break ups, or friendships that suddenly ended. Maybe even friend groups that began to turn on us or careers that seem to be against us. Everyone would experience the natural necessary sadness of these experiences. However, as we begin to ruminate on the past and worry about them repeating in the future, we may find ourselves blaming ourselves over our past actions or even shaming ourselves about who we were / are (i.e., *"I am unlovable... I am a failure.... I'm cursed!"*). Thus, making us depressed and full of shame, which may perpetuate the cycle of separating ourselves more and more from the reality *"as it is."* In doing this we are activating the destructiveness of the separate self that is judgemental, non-accepting, and refusing to let go of others' transgressions, and thereby our own. The difficulty of course is that as we go farther down this well, it becomes darker and harder to find the light. One way to shine a light is through acceptance without judgement that the past has passed.

"As we continue to live in the reality as we want it to be, we sit and wait in the well for help. We believe it is getting darker & darker, both externally and internally. However, only by non-judgementally accepting reality as it is can we begin to look upward and find the light of self-compassion with its peace and true lasting happiness."

NAIL A BET: A Mindful Tool for Emotional Healing

Introduction

As previously mentioned, NAIL is a powerful mindfulness technique that can be used to observe our emotional experiences (i.e., an Emotional Check In) so that we can learn from them. However, the advance version allows us to choose between investigating and learning from it or simply de-identifying from the stimuli and letting go of destructive emotions. The more often we practice this, the easier it gets. NAIL A BET is the advanced version of this. Described below is a therapeutic tool designed to guide individuals through the mindful processing of *B*ody sensations, *E*motions, and *T*houghts (BETs). This tool integrates 10 factors across 4 steps, with a focus on cultivating awareness and compassion to dissolve the harmful energy of challenging emotions. By conducting the NAIL A BET process one can prevent the Cyclic Self-Destructive pattern we all face and instead maintain a path toward well-being.

The Four Steps of NAIL A BET

1. **Notice Non-judgmentally (N) in the Here and Now**
   The first step involves holding the energy of body sensations, emotions, and thoughts (BETs) in the mind, focusing on noticing these experiences in the here and Now of the present moment without judgement. "N" stands for both noticing, but more importantly, noticing non-judgmentally. This encourages you to bring your full attention to what is happening right now versus what you think will be in the future, or assuming what happened before in the past will happen now.

2. **Accept and Allow (A)**
   In the second step, the focus shifts to accepting and allowing the experiences noticed in the first step. Acceptance here does not mean resignation, but rather an open and non-judgmental acknowledgment of whatever is present in the mind and body. This step is crucial for creating a space where these experiences can be fully felt without using the three avoidances of ignoring, indulging and rejecting.

3. **Investigate and Non-Identification (I)**
   The third step involves investigating the experiences with mindful curiosity while avoiding identification with whatever is coming up for you. This means observing the BETs without labeling them as "yours" or attaching to them. This allows you to see the BET as temporary and not as part of who you are.

4. **Learn, Let it Come, Let Be, Let Go (L)**
   The final step is multifaceted, incorporating four important actions:

   - **Learn** about the impermanent, imperfect, and impersonal nature of reality, often referred to as *"the way it is."*

   - **Let** the energy of BETs fully come into awareness without resistance.

   - **Let** them be just as they are, without trying to change or control them.

   - **Let** them go, allowing the energy of these experiences to dissipate naturally through mindful compassion, meaning feeling the energy of a BET complex with no added thinking.

Compassionately NAIL A BET

The "A" in NAIL A BET stands for awareness, which serves as the underlying approach throughout the process. By applying mindful awareness with compassion, individuals can shortcut the lengthy process of traditional meditation. This method offers a structured yet flexible approach to dealing with the core emotions / experiences of Anger, Addictiveness, Apathy, Anxiety, and Ambivalence and the derivative affective states of shame, guilt, remorse, & pride. These affective states are important to know because they are the mind factors that will distract you as you try to mindfully shift towards wellness.

What is a BET complex?

The three components of this complex don't occur alone but follow Law 6 of Connectivity (Figure 1 on page 5), such that they are all connected to each other and work together. For example, for every angry thought is a connected body sensation like tight muscles and emotions of anger. What they share is a common destructive energy, which is what you feel and should be what you mindfully experience with compassion to dissolve away.

Preventing Cyclic Self-Destructive Behavior

The first three steps of NAIL A BET prepare the mind to engage with the final step, where the focus is on letting go. Through mindful compassion, the harmful energy associated with these emotional states can be dissolved, preventing them from being stored in the body and mind. This approach helps individuals avoid the path of Cyclic Self-Destructiveness and instead maintain a trajectory toward well-being.

NAIL A BET is a practical and effective tool for those seeking to manage and transform difficult emotions. By following its four steps individuals can cultivate a deeper understanding of their emotional experiences and dissolve the harmful energy that often leads to self-destructive behaviors. This mindful approach not only aids in emotional healing but also supports long-term well-being by keeping individuals on a positive path, free from the cycles of suffering that can arise from unprocessed emotional energy.

Exercise for Week #2: NAIL A BET in One's Body & Mind

The first goal is to continue 15-20 minutes of daily meditation. The meditation this week will focus on scanning one's <u>B</u>ody sensations learning to accept them as they are, temporary and non-personal, so that you can learn to let them go along with their associated <u>E</u>motions and <u>T</u>houghts, thus in the process the complete BET complex.

Theory of Body Scan Meditation

1. Simply become aware of your body from head to toe noticing any sensations that may come to your Mind.
2. Don't try to change what you are experiencing. Become aware of the feeling, and just experience it non-judgmentally.
3. Your goal is to be aware, accept, and allow just as you did previously with your breathing.
4. Notice the body sensations come, be and go, as well as the connecting emotions or thoughts.
5. You do this to learn that all things are connected and have a beginning, middle, and end.

"Allow your body sensations to reveal the truth of health & happiness that is being hidden from thinking distorted by emotions."

After reading through the above theory, practice the below steps once per day. Learn to Notice Non-judgementally and accept your body's sensations as they are versus the way you want them to.

Steps to Body Scan Meditation (*From Puhalla & Puhalla, 2023*)

1. Start in any comfortable position, standing, sitting, or lying.

2. Breathe deeply with the intention you will be *calm yet alert, accepting and kind*, to develop increasing levels of single focused concentration.

3. Begin by bringing awareness to your body. Start from your feet, moving up towards your head, or do it from head to toe.

4. At each body part, notice what you feel there, for it may be holding the energy of a destructive emotion.

5. Continue scanning through your entire body. Pay attention to where you're holding tension, to areas of pain, pressure, or tightness.

6. Stay continuously focused with the sensation revealing its emotion.

7. When you find that sensation-emotion, notice what accompanying thoughts you may be having.

8. Make a connection with the body sensation. For example, say it is tight neck muscles with an emotion, like anger, and thoughts, like, *"work is frustrating."*

9. For now, these thoughts are distractions, that once noticed you store in the back of your mind, for future contemplation.

10. After you have given the thoughts some brief kind attention, without adding further thoughts, return to feeling the sensation-emotion.

11. Don't avoid feeling the emotion, like anger, but feel it from beginning to its end, so it is dissolved away and in the future you will know that if you are having that body sensation you know it is related to anger.

12. To mindfully dissolve this energy, apply the healing power of compassion directed both to yourself and all others. Do this with each passing breath.

13. Take in sensations with the in breath, and let troublesome associated emotions go, with the out breath. For example, in breath, feel the stiff neck muscles, with the out breath, let go of the associated destructive anger, doing this over and over, will dissolve away both the discomfort of the stiff neck muscles and the destructiveness of the angry emotions' energy and associated harmful thinking.

14. Repeat this cycle for 10-20 minutes using your breath or the instructions as anchor.

Remember, just in scanning the body, continuously focusing on one body part at a time, you are developing mindfulness. As you learn to naturally dissolve the unwanted sensations and destructive emotions during the exercise, you are also learning to become more compassionate towards yourself. Overtime, this will extend to when you are not meditating, which may allow you to quickly evaluate where you are holding your emotions and dissolve them before they are stored.

Steps to Acceptance Based Imagery

Similar to the deep breathing exercise, individuals who have strong visualization may benefit from using guided or self-guided imagery. Below are basic instructions on how to attempt guided imagery based on the same principle. Apply these steps after a few minutes of deep breathing to get yourself focused, calm, and alert. Don't forget in all of these trainings to do them with an attitude of kindness and acceptance of *"the way it is."*

1. Slowly begin to visualize a flowing river or rapid. This can be a real river or one that you made only in your mind's eye.

2. Visualize the passing of the water and the ripples of the water rushing past, as if they are your very own emotions, thoughts, and memories about the past.

3. You may also visualize the scenery around the lake if it helps you become aware of the rapid nature of your mental energy.

4. As you observe the river continue to slow your breathing. Try with time to make it slower and slower.

5. Now imagine that the rapids, and quick moving water are specific thoughts, emotions, and physical sensations from the past and future that keep getting stuck in a natural dam.

6. Visualize the dam as the separate self that wishes to hold on to the past.

7. Visualize these BETs as all running into the dam of non-acceptance as you breath in.

8. With each exhale imagine the natural dam opening to see that the BETs are temporary and will pass by.

9. Leave the dam open to accept the river as it is, which represents the constant flowing of one's mind and mental energy.

10. Return to your breath as needed to continue with the visualization.

11. Repeat the cycle above repeatedly until the river becomes free flowing.

Each day conduct 15-20 minutes of meditative practice to strengthen your ability to accept reality as it is. Additionally, each day complete NAIL A BET and document the experience (see figure 5).

Figure 5. **NAIL A BET LOG**

Notice-Non-Judgmentally	Accept as it is	Investigate or De-Identify	Learn & Let Go
Feeling depressed	It is just a moment of sadness	I miss loved ones, but this is just a momentary thought not who I permanently am	This will pass, just like all emotions. Focus on what I have control over.

3. Holding On to the Past Only Drains

Weighted down by the memories of yesterday so we cannot grow today

"What has happened in the past has passed. Let it go and accept it as it is, so you can live in the here and now instead of the way you wished it could have been."

Mirror 3 - A Mirror holds onto nothing, so it cannot be weighed down

Just like a mirror, the connected compassionate self does not hold onto the past, as it does not overly identify with past successes or failures, joyful or sorrowful moments, or any other moment of time that may pull us to the past to try and make it *"the way we want it to be."* Instead, the connected compassionate self provides gentle kindness towards its perceived past self and forgives itself for what did not go *"to plan"* and doesn't overly attach to prideful moments. This allows for one to both enjoy the memories of the past, without assuming that they will repeat themselves. By overly holding onto the past one can become weighted down by it and find themselves focused either on (a) attempting to preserve it (if it positive) or (b) attempting to change it or "disprove" it (i.e., trying to change the past). This is different than mindfully examining our past behaviors to grow from them, as these BETs often occur without thought.

"A Mirror by its nature holds on to nothing, letting everything fully come, fully be, just as it is, so it can let all of its energy fully go."

This separate self that is attempting to preserve (i.e., overly indulge) or reject the past will also attempt to do that in the here and now.

It can be as simple as attempting to continue to be "perceived" as something we no longer are, or as something completely new as we have not let go of the past to be completely present in the here and now.

For example, many individuals who experience physical or sexual assault can find themselves attempting to mask their feelings of fear or anxiety in social / dating situations by coming off as bold, direct, or even hostile / aggression. This pattern, along with the flip, are both examples of holding onto the past out of desires to change it into the way they wished it could have been.

To learn to let go of the past, one must learn to be kind, empathetic, and forgiving to their past self. By learning that all BETs are impermanent (i.e., always flowing), imperfect (i.e., are usually not the complete "facts"), and impersonal (i.e., even our own thoughts are not our own) one can begin this process by no longer staying in the cycle of unnecessary suffering via rejecting the negatives, overindulging the positives, and ignoring the neutral moments. By first meditating and then engaging in contemplation meditation on the three Is (i.e., imperfection, impermanence, and impersonal nature of BETs) we can place our past selves in better contextual understanding to begin to de-attach from it so we can begin to accept the past and present as it is.

"It's attachment to an independent self-view that separates us from the truth, others, and humaneness, resulting in feeling lost, lonely, and lacking, leading to a despairing existential depression"

Exercise for Week #3: Learn to Let it Go One Breath at a Time

First we must be present so that we can accept *"the way it is,"* but to continue doing this for ourselves, others, and all those we love we must learn to let go of the separate self that wants us to hold onto to the past and desire to change it to *"the way we want it to be."* To do this, continue practicing 15-20 minutes of meditation per day. No additional exercises besides the breathing and imagery-based meditations will be provided this week, however, continue to use NAIL A BET as needed.

Let it Come, Let it Be, Let it Go Meditation

One of the simplest ways to meditate is to apply the Let it come, be, & go principles to the desires of attachment of the past and present being the way *"you want it to be"* so you can begin living in the reality as it is.

Step 1: Let it Come: Become aware of your breathing, feeling its sensation, focusing on the in breath. Feel it coming from beginning to end.

Step 2: Let it Be: As you are letting the breath fully come, don't interfere with it by changing or controlling, or comparing it to past breaths, or wanting something, and expectation from it, just let it be, as it is accepted fully. If you are controlling, changing, comparing or expecting, you are thinking and not being mindful. Notice this, and go back to feeling the breathing.

Step 3: Let it Go: After the in breath reaches its peak, and you notice the pause, you are now ready to let it go, noticing and feeling the going away process from its beginning to its end, and noticing the pause.

Meditation: Let it Come, Be & Go with Compassionate Forgiveness

1. Repeat these three steps over and over, following the natural flow of your breathing, without thinking, staying in the present, with kindness and full acceptance and not judging.

2. Find the breath, feeling its flow, free of any thinking to stay single and continuously focused on the breath.

3. When you are distracted by anything, notice it with kind forgiveness, with no self-judgment, accepting this as a natural part of meditation.

4. The mind automatically creates thoughts, do not add further thoughts, but just watch their energy come and go.

5. If you do add additional thoughts to create a new reality, just gently focus on them and accept them as impermanent, imperfect, and impersonal. With the next exhale, let them go and forgive yourself for being distracted; it is normal and to be expected to have automatic distractions of a BET, notice it, accept it, observe it, let it go, over & over.

6. Letting it go is watching and experiencing natural energy burning away, until it is completely gone, like watching a fire burn itself out.

7. Repeat this process over and over, instilling greater amounts of compassion and forgiveness with each distraction. Focus on cultivating compassion within you to learn to let go of the weight of the idea that anyone can be perfect. Accept everyone is perfectly imperfect.

Steps to Letting Go Based Imagery

Below are basic instructions on how to attempt guided imagery based on the same principle. Always begin with about 5 minutes of deep breathing to first become focused. Apply these steps after a few minutes of deep breathing to get yourself focused, calm, and alert.

1. Slowly begin to visualize a sunny, but cloudy sky above you.

2. Imagine the hints of blue, and the assorted colors of the clouds.

3. If possible, even imagine the feeling of the sun raining rays of light upon you, as well as the gentle wind whisking by.

4. Now imagine that each memory of the past or about yourself is a new cloud. With smaller clouds representing small BETs, while large darker clouds are deeper, and darker thoughts of yourself and the past.

5. As you observe the clouds continue to slow your breathing. Try with time to make it slower and slower.

6. Now imagine that the sun is the connected compassionate self beginning to dissolve away the clouds.

7. Allow each cloud to naturally dissolve away from the forgiving nature of the light of the sun and return to the gentle view of the sunny sky.

8. Return to your breath as needed to continue with the visualization.

9. Sooner or later other BETs you want to hold onto will come up.

10. Repeat the above process.

Each day, conduct 15-20 minutes of meditation to strengthen your ability to let go of the reality as the way you want it to be, so you can instill greater compassion and feelings of connection for yourself and your loved ones. Please use figure 6 to reflect on this practice.

Figure 6. Meditation Log

Date	Meditation Type	What BETs distracted you the most?	How can you instill greater compassion next practice?

4. Self-Love for Self-Growth

Love yourself first, and others will follow

"Loving yourself does not mean giving in to avoidance and focusing on the separate self, but embracing the compassionate connected self"

Mirror 4: Love can only Reflect Love

We attract not what we want, but what energy we put into the world (Law 2), and this energy will comes back to us in return (Law 1), but only in its own time (Law 11). As such, only through self-growth (Law 3) can we begin to find kindness, warmth, forgiveness, and compassion. By instilling these highest of virtues towards oneself they eventually will be returned too, so it is especially important to practice loving-kindness and compassion towards our own mistakes and negative BETs.

Always stay aware of you BETs as body sensations, especially of pains and discomforts, emotions especially of worry, sadness, anger, shame and guilt, and the energy of your negative thoughts so you can deal with them in the present. Accept them, and let them go, so you grow in love and compassion.

To activate the Compassionate Connected Self, one must learn to let go of separate self, as the separate self's goal is to preserve the reality *"as it wants it to be,"* versus *"the way it is."* What this means is that even if we say we are trying to be kind and understanding to other people, if we prioritize maintaining our own reality then we will do almost anything to preserve it. This is what leads to the selfishness of the separate self.

We will engage in greed and hateful action, for the sake of "protecting" ourselves or what we identify with. Of course, there are times we must be assertive and allow natural anger to occur.

However, as the majority of threat is no longer life or integrity threat, it means many of the times we believe we must "protect ourselves" it is ego threat towards the separate self. Comparatively, Selfless Love, even towards oneself, does not misinform, but always reflects the wholesome truth of reality. It keeps oneself and others in the present, with a single focus on accepting reality as it is. In this, the priority is towards the highest levels of health, happiness, and a peacefulness. Doing this will keep you on the path of the reflections of this mirror of Selfless Connected Love.

Meditation and daily acts of compassion can begin a journey towards this. By being present with yourself through meditation you can clean your mind of false belief of the separate self, greed, & hate, that no matter how small, have accidently attracted people who misinform, are greedy, and hateful.

Thus, selfless love reflects to us Courage in the face of anxiety, Compassion when anger wants to overcome us, a Centred balanced wanting or not wanting when we want to overly indulge in addictive pleasures, Caring intentions when we feel a sense of apathy of depression, & Certainty in the face of unknown future (i.e., the 5 Cs of compassion).

For example, many people with severe anxiety or PTSD can find themselves in a positive feedback loop between avoidance and negatives BETs through rejecting negatives (e.g., not leaving the house to go shopping out of fear), ignoring neutrals (e.g., always distracting oneself out of fear of what might enter their mind), and over indulging in positives (e.g., over consuming alcohol or cannabis to sooth negative emotions and induce positive ones beyond a healthy level).

This entire loop is to preserve the reality as *"the way the anxiety / PTSD wants it to be."* By no direct choice in oneself, this creates a self-destructive process that can leave individuals feeling severely depressed, feeling disconnected from loved ones, without the ability to be the authors of their own lives.

By meditating and engaging in daily acts of compassion, with no additional goal of gain besides putting positive energy into the world, individuals with severe anxiety, PTSD, and depression can also learn to cultivate the compassionate connected self.

For example, when one wants to avoid going to the store to shop for their family, out of fear of what could happen, they can mediate on Courage of what it would mean to be able to feed themselves and their family, even in the face of anxiety.

If you notice you become quickly angry at someone who cuts you off on the road or is rude to you in a hallway, then engage in Compassionate understanding to see / feel what they feel (e.g., *"The person who cut you off may have an illness, may be rushing to pick up their child from a program, may be someone's grandmother, and etc."*).

Finally, instead of over-indulging in sensory pleasures like alcohol or drugs to "feel good," build a Centred practice around self-care that can be conducted every day (e.g., small treat at the end of the day, exercise time, listening to your favorite music, and etc...).

Anger, hatred, and revenge is like attempting to poison another, but often we end up drinking the poison ourselves. Learning to be compassionate, even towards those we have neutral or negative feelings towards, will only cultivate greater compassion towards oneself in the end. For example, blaring one's horn after another driver puts you in danger may "feel" like it is in your best interest, however, after the safety concern is over, it is only putting stress on your own body and toxic energy into the environment (i.e., the continuous blaring of the horn). Instead, letting go of the energy, with the above techniques, will put less strain on your mind, body, and the environment. In fact, it may even put positive emotions and energy into the world.

Use figure 7, a contrast of the Separate & Compassionate Self, to contemplate the experiences, advantages & disadvantages of the choice to either attract the qualities of a separate versus connected self, & its false selfish love vs true selfless love.

Figure 7. The Separate Self vs. The Connected Self

Seperate Self	Connected Self
☐ "way you want it to be"	☐ "the way it really is,"
☐ Motivated by desire	☐ Humane motivations
☐ Desire is never Satisfied	☐ Humaneness is satisfaction
☐ Avoidance causes distress	☐ Acceptance as stress relief
☐ Hold on to pleasure	☐ Satisfaction is letting go
☐ Satisfaction is outside	☐ Satisfaction in the Mind
☐ Avoid pain to harm	☐ Take in Pain to Help
☐ Judgemental biased	☐ Accepts all equally
☐ Progressive anger	☐ Kind patient peaceful
☐ Un-caring to suffering	☐ Altruistic compassion
☐ Illness Ageing Death	☐ Health HappinessPeace
☐ Avoid to Cycle Suffering	☐ Acceptance ends suffering

Exercise for Week #4: Fostering Self-love

Continue to practice meditation each day for 15-20 minutes. Breathing meditation, or any of its variants we have introduced, all are useful to have a singular focus or one item to concentrate on. However, one of the additional goals of meditation is to begin contemplating or mindfully exploring specific topics for self-growth. As such, this week we will begin to cultivate loving-kindness through a Loving-Kindness meditation. Similar to all the other exercises, you will become distracted and that is okay! That is part of the learning process. Return to your breath to recenter yourself and continue with the meditation, over and over.

Loving Kindness Meditation

Similar to all other meditations, start with about 5 minutes of deep breathing meditation to help you become focused. Utilize the ABC-Ds of breathing meditation to help with this and remember, *"breath, breath, distract, & repeat."* The below instructions are for after this period.

1. First notice the sensation of your breath as you breathe in and out.

2. Notice the positive energy of life as you breathe in, and letting go of any negative energy as you breathe out.

3. Next begin by sending loving-kindness towards ourselves by sending positive intentions inwards. Gently say out loud or internally:
    a. *May I be kind towards myself.*
    b. *May I be forgiving towards myself.*
    c. *May I extend the same empathy I send to my love ones to myself.*
    d. *May I find the patience I need in the here and now.*
    e. *May I find the courage to persevere through the natural suffering of life.*
    f. *May I find the compassionate understanding that I need.*

Creating Compassion

4. Continue with your slow, deep, and controlled breathing.

5. Focus on whatever loving intention that you need as you focus on your breath. Cultivate that intention and observe the physical sensations that you experience.

6. Do you notice a sense a warmth? Maybe a sense of expansion outwards? Or a desire to smile, laugh, or even cry? Whatever that sensation is allow it to be, just as it is, and remain present for it.

7. Now we will extend this loving-kindness towards someone you care about in your life.

8. This may be a partner, parent, child, friend, or pet. Whoever you believe needs this right now.

9. Send these positive intentions towards them by gently saying out loud or internally:
    a. *May I send you the kindness that you need.*
    b. *May you find the forgiveness for the past and present.*
    c. *May you feel heard and seen by those around you.*
    d. *May I be with you patiently throughout your journey.*
    e. *May you find the courage you need to persevere.*
    f. *May you find the compassionate understand that we all need.*

10. Continue with your slow, deep, and controlled breathing.

11. Focus on whatever loving intention that you most want to send to them.

Creating Compassion

12. Do you notice a sense of warmth? Maybe a sense of expansion outwards? Or a desire to smile, laugh, or even cry? Whatever that sensation is allow it to be, just as it is, and remain present for it.

13. Now we will extend this loving-kindness towards all living beings.

14. Send these positive intentions towards all living beings by gently saying out loud or internally:
    a. *May I send you all the kindness that you need.*
    b. *May you all find the forgiveness you need for the past and present.*
    c. *May all feel heard and seen by those around you.*
    d. *May we all find the patience to allow the journey to naturally be*
    e. *May we all find the courage we need to persevere.*
    f. *May you all find the compassionate understand that we all need.*

15. Continue with your slow, deep, and controlled breathing.

16. Focus on whatever loving intention that you need the most right now.

17. Notice the energy it brings to you.

18. Gently place your hand over your heart and internally or gently out loud say the intention you need the most right now.

19. Repeat this process or allow yourself to gently return to present moment.

Steps to Loving Kindness Imagery

Apply these steps after a few minutes of deep breathing to get yourself focused, calm, and alert. Don't forget in all of these trainings to do them with an attitude of kindness and acceptance of *"the way it is."*

1. Slowly begin to visualize a place of pure warmth and brightness. This can be a real place or one of the mind's creation. Imagine the details of the location.

2. The location may be a warm beach, or a cabin with light rays pouring in from outside.

3. It may be a church, temple, or place of religious importance.

4. Or it could be a simple place where light is raining in that makes you feel connected to the universe.

5. As you observe the light rays pouring into this location, notice as they naturally expand and contract with each inhale and exhale.

6. Sooner or later, you will be distracted. Just return to the warming experience of this imagery.

7. Visualize the warmth of the rays of light slowly melting away any negative emotions you may be experiencing.

8. With each exhale allow the warm, love, and compassion of the light to dissolve one's anger towards oneself and others.

9. Return to your breath as needed to continue with the visualization.

10. If you notice resentment, anger, shame, or guilt, over a current or past action, allow the light to gently fold around the emotion or memory.

11. After it surrounds the BET, slowly let it dissolve the emotional experience as you return to feeling the warm embrace of the light.

12. Repeat this process and allow any natural emotions to come, be, and go.

13. Thank yourself for the meditative experience at the end.

Practice one, or both, of these loving kindness meditations <u>each day</u> along with breath work. Notice any judgements about yourself that you make and attempt to return to the exercise with the same patience, kindness, compassion and forgiveness you would give to your closest loved one.

If Selfless love comes from focusing on self-growth, then we need to focus on behavioural actions of self-love / self-kindness. This does not mean overindulging, or spending money, but instead spending time on oneself in the here and now. Each day, attempt to engage in one act of self-compassion / self-love. This can be as simple as listening to music while drinking your morning coffee, or going for a walk while listening to a podcast. Whatever you notice you *"don't have time for,"* make time for it.

Experience these moments mindfully without judgement (e.g., *"ahhh, I should be checking emails instead of drinking this coffee and listening to this music.... [during exercise] ughhh I am not nearly as strong as I use to be [or] as fast as I use to be"*). If you notice judgements come, then use NAIL A BET and let them go. These moments of kindness can be shared with loved ones and are highly recommended to be shared (see figure 8).

Figure 8. Loving-Kindness Meditation & Action Log

Date	Meditation Type	Loving-Kindness Action	What Judgements or BETs came up?

5. Create the Joy You Seek

Kindness & Compassion will be returned… In its own time.

"Happiness & satisfaction does not come from over indulgence and luxury, but from self-growth via the compassionate connected self"

Mirror 5 of Creation - A Mirror Creates a Truthful Reflection.

A question asked over and over again, is why am I not happy if I am "successful?" It comes simply down to the notion that success, however it is conceptualized, is impermeant, impersonal, and imperfect. In other words, all types of success (e.g.., financial, interpersonal, professional, & etc.) will have ebbs and flows and basing our happiness on it will lead to attachment to the moments that we deemed as successful and thus living a reality *"as we want it to be."* Additionally, success is not just ours, but all that led to it, so over attachment to it is inaccurate in nature, as there are many factors that determine success.

Finally, the more success one finds the more they can find wrong in that success. In careers it can be a higher pay check after a promotion, or a more prestigious / important position. In relationships it can be getting married or having a connected relationship with one's family, but then we become concerned about how our relationships "appear" to others. Thus, leaving us wanting for more and more, establishing greater attachment to success, and attempting to find ways to maintain it, even if it is only in name.

The separate self can push us well beyond the normative pattern of unnecessary suffering and desires for more. The separate self can lead to dramatic issues when we deem ourselves "unsuccessful," as over time we may hold onto this image of ourselves which can skew the reality *"as it is"* more and more into what the separate self wants it to be.

For example, the individual who bases their worth on their job and how much money they make can find themselves focusing on the gains / fame of their career and the admiration that their family, friends, and colleagues provide them for their success. If this is the case, then an individual may disregard the level of stress the job causes or pay too much attention to their work over their family. This can lead to severe anxiety or dread over work, as they feel they "must" maintain this level of success or they may be perceived as a "failure," or "fraud."

As these fears of being perceived as something one believes they are not escalate, it can cause a spiral of negative self-talk when work doesn't go well in an attempt to hold onto the identity of being "successful." Instead, we need to active the compassionate connected self to accept reality *"as it is"* and seeing each moment in any one domain of one's life as temporary, imperfect, and impersonal. After accepting reality *"as it is,"* we then must ask what is not just in the best interest of the superficial self, but our mind, body, and for all others.

"What's done for others, motivated by lasting Humane Values, of kindness, sharing, acceptance & compassion, lives on forever in the mind of all others."

To do this we want to continue to cultivate the highest humane virtues. By cultivating the highest humane virtues, you are transmitting compassion from yourself to all other beings, which will return to you in its own time.

Modern day wants us to be focus on self-serving pursuits, but this will only lead to temporary happiness. Instead focus on intentions of kindness, sharing, acceptance, & compassion to have lasting happiness and a peaceful mind. Over time, this will become easier as you get use to NAIL(ing) A BET and refocusing on the underlying intentions of the highest humane values.

"Let go a little to be a little happy, let go a lot, be a lot happy, let go of everything all the time, holding on to nothing & you will be at Peace."

Highest Humane Values

There are many definitions of these highest humane values, with several books well equipped at assisting people in understanding loving-kindness meditation (e.g., Gunaratana, 2017). Below are some basic definitions that can be the focus of contemplative meditation.

1. **Kindness**: To deeply know so you can care for oneself, all others, and things.

2. **Equanimity**: Learn to accept all things equally. Accept all experiences with yourself, others, and all beings, regardless if they are positive, negative, or neutral, equally. Allow all energy to come, be, and go.

3. **Sympathetic Joy:** Enjoy positivity with all others with no envy.

4. **Compassion**: To altruistically engage with all beings in the hopes to end all unnecessary suffering.

These virtues can act as antidotes to everyday unnecessary suffering, as when we apply them to anxiety, anger, apathy, and addictive desire they can help them dissolve away and thereby dissolve the depression within. However, to do this we must cultivate each virtue in contemplation meditation and in daily action.

Four Worldly Desires

These four humane values are not only antidotes for success, but for the four worldly desires of any pleasure without pain, gain without loss, credits without blames, and fame without infamy.

These also cause conflict because we want the pleasure without it eventually passing away to result in pain, the same for wanting gain without loss, credits without blames, and fame without infamy. This happens because the Separate Self cannot accept these with their impermanence, for it would weaken the perception of the Self as permanent.

Remember the Separate Self loves itself, at the expense of the rest of the mind, the body, all others, and the needs of the outside world. To love one's self is to love all of one's connections. With compassion you must feel the loss of pleasures becoming pains, as they occur, and the impermanence of the other three desires, so you don't add distress to the stress of life's losses, which will diminish your self-love, and that which you then share with others.

Exercise for Week #5: Build the Compassion You Seek

To be able to enjoy the moment with oneself and others, without jealousy or desire, one needs to learn to forgive oneself for their own imperfection. The great news is, we can always practice this during meditation. Follow the steps below to learn greater self-forgiveness.

First practice it within meditation, then day-to-day life, and then finally with deeper components of yourself. Similar to the previous exercises, attempt to meditate 15-20 minutes per day in whatever increments that are realistic for you.

Creating Compassion

Meditation on Radical Acceptance:

1. Begin by sitting in a centered, balanced, and stable stance. This may include sitting on the floor or in a chair, but make sure you are stable so that you will not need to keep correcting your posture. Additionally, if the posture is too relaxed, make sure you balance it with an upright posture to remain attentive.

2. Focus on your breath following the ABC-Ds of deep breathing.

3. Become aware of breath and concentrate only on that.

4. Focus on the sensation as you breath in and out.

5. You will become distracted, but just observe the distraction and let it go with your next exhale.

6. Once centered, begin to notice your distractions with a new purpose.

7. Instead of simply letting them go or being pulled away by them, observe why you are so bothered by them.

8. Is it because you believe you are beyond distraction?

9. Is it because you are bored and rather pay attention to something else?

10. Is it because you are having a future desire?

11. Or maybe the distraction of sleepiness or pain?

12. Forgive yourself over and over again for this distraction, even verbalizing it if you need to.

13. Repeat this cycle: Breath, Breath, Distracted, Forgive, & Repeat!

Radical Acceptance Imagery Exercise:

1. Begin by conducting 5 minutes of deep breathing meditation.

2. Once centered, begin to visualize yourself hiking up a mountain. Visualize the plants and wildlife around you.

3. Imagine the temperature and the feeling of pushing yourself along the trail.

4. Try your best to see in your mind's eye the path in front of you.

5. With each inhale imagine going further and further up the mountain side.

6. Now imagine you have a backpack with you that is heavy.

7. The items in the backpack represent your past memories, future worries / wants, and current distractors.

8. With each BET that enters your mind, imagine that it is an item that is weighing you down in your bag.

9. With your next exhale imagine taking that BET out of your bag and forgiving yourself for carrying it this long before you let it go.

10. Continue along the path with your next inhale.

11. Repeat this process over and over again until you freed of the past that is weighing you down so you can visualize and travel up this mountain trail.

To create the kindness, forgiveness, equality, and compassion one seeks, then we must put it into the world towards ourselves and others. Continue engaging in daily loving-kindness actions and logging what judgements or BETs get in the way. Have these moments with yourself and others and log what got in the way of forgiving yourself when they were not perfect.

Figure 9. Loving-Kindness Meditation & Action Log

Date	Meditation Type	Loving-Kindness Action (Towards self? Shared with others?)	What Judgements got in the way? Were you able to forgive & let go?

6. Unification versus Separation

Living in a state of extremes will only return extremes.

"Unify through connection & compassion to dissolve anger and despair"

Mirror 6 -Unification of the extremes

Based on basic cognitive theory, we all learn to categorize the world around us through language. As early as toddlerhood we begin to specify what is a dog versus a cat, a chair versus a table, and then (eventually) what is good versus bad. As we get older, we become aware that urges, actions, and morals are not that simple. Yet, we continue to utilize *"all or none"* or extreme thinking that is based on dualism.

- Good vs. Bad
- Right vs. Wrong
- Happiness vs. Suffering
- Healthy vs. Damaging
- Survival vs. Death

The solution to dualistic thinking is making a choice to change from "either-or" to "neither-nor." For example, in happiness vs. suffering, one would think that in happiness is already suffering, and in suffering there is happiness. If you experience happiness, you will find as it passes away there is suffering, that must be experienced with compassion so you don't add distress to the stress of this loss. This distress is added unnecessary suffering.

In regard to dissolving unnecessary suffering, we must learn to radically accept and provide kindness to our basic human instincts that, when left unobserved, can encourage dualistic thinking and thereby add unnecessary suffering through avoidance.

For example, it is in our basic nature to strive to survive and flourish and create a system where our most immediate loved ones do as well.

However, when we engage in dualistic thinking with these ends in mind we can become blinded by all or none / extreme thinking that can lead to unnecessary suffering.

For example, when a friend or loved one insults you or says something that hurts your feelings, then you may take in personally, believe it is (perfectly) accurate, and maintain the negative emotions privately.

Thus, one difficult moment is extended by internalized shame from that individual. It could also turn into anger towards them if you find what they say as being inaccurate as you attempt to continue to preserve the reality *as you want it to be.* Comparatively, if a stranger or an acquaintance insults you, then you may be quick to anger towards them and even engage in aggressive behavior (e.g., Cursing at them, engaging in lude behavior, or returning an insult yourself). In both situations unnecessary suffering is added, at least, to yourself if not to other people.

By seeing that all energy falls on a spectrum and learning to respond to it with kindness & curiosity one can learn to dissolve these negative emotions and not extend suffering. In fact, in the former example, learning to observe your emotional reaction and responding with assertiveness, with a gentle tone, may be the most kind thing to do for yourself and your loved one.

Comparatively, what good comes from becoming angry and aggressive towards the stranger? It may momentarily preserve your reality *as you want it to be*, but over time that anger and negative energy will extend towards yourself and those you care about either directly (e.g., becoming a more hostile individual in general) or indirectly (e.g., high blood pressure, heart disease, & etc.). Thus, the goal is to acknowledge and let go of our <u>Human</u> animal instincts, besides when we are in life threatening situations, and cultivate our highest <u>Humane values</u>.

"Because of the false beliefs of dualistic thinking we are blinded to our Mind's true complete nature and we add suffering to living ."

To remove this dualistic thinking requires us to radically accept the reality *"as it is"* versus the *"the way we want it to be."* None of us want to be angry, fearful, jealous individuals. However, we all have moments when these natural emotions occur and automatic reactions follow. To engage in further self-growth, the second step after radically accepting the emotional experience *"as it is"* must be pausing before we automatically respond again. From there we have already broken the loop that we often are stuck in and then can make a choice towards our deeper values.

Thus, the goal of this mirror is to unify Humane values with your Human instinctual qualities. This means being sure of the following:

To avoid adding unnecessary suffering be sure that "the way I want it be" accurately represents "the way it is."

By applying the light of awareness & understanding we can remove the unnecessary attachment to our BETs, which over time will reduce unnecessary suffering. After this we can focus on cultivating kindness, generosity, warmth, and forgiveness to ourselves and others instead of just *reacting* (a.k.a. single focus).

"If the goal is being humanely peaceful, it's energy must be unified with the experience of temporary suffering of the inevitable losses."

To help with cultivating the Compassionate Self through unification of our natural reactions and humane values, ask yourself one or multiple of these questions each day during meditative practice. You can also choose to write about these.

Questions to Contemplate for Unifying Wholesome Choices

1. Identifying the Cycle of Separation:

1. Am I ignoring aspects of my life that cause discomfort or challenge my sense of self?

2. Do I find myself constantly grasping for things I desire, even when they may not be helpful?

3. Am I avoiding situations or emotions that make me uncomfortable, rather than facing them?

4. Do I often identify my emotions as being a core part of who I am?

5. Am I obsessively thinking about things that have happened or might happen, unable to let go?

6. Do I feel compelled to constantly do something to avoid uncomfortable feelings?

7. Do I feel isolated or disconnected from others, believing that I am separate and alone?

8. Do I prioritize my own needs and desires over those of others, even when it causes harm?

9. Do I feel a constant craving for more, never feeling satisfied with what I have?

10. Do I see myself as a fixed, unchanging entity, unable to adapt to new situations?

11. Do I perceive the world as hostile or threatening, believing that it is against me?

12. Do I act out of desperation or anger, often leading to violent or harmful behavior?

2. Identifying steps towards Unification?

1. Am I staying aware of the present moment and the reality of my situation?
2. Am I able to let go of my desires when they do not serve my well-being?
3. Am I accepting the way things are, rather than resisting it?
4. Do I see my emotions as transient energies, rather than identifying with them as who I am?
5. Am I able to observe my thoughts mindfully, without getting caught up in them?
6. Can I stay still and reflective, even in the face of discomfort or uncertainty?
7. Do I feel connected to others, understanding that we are all part of a greater whole?
8. Do I act with selflessness, prioritizing compassionate actions for the benefit of all?
9. Am I content with what I have, finding satisfaction in the present moment?
10. Do I understand that my sense of self is fluid and ever-changing, adapting to new realities?
11. Do I perceive the world with compassion and wisdom, seeking to understand rather than judge?
12. Do I respond to challenges with kindness and calm, rather than with fear or anger?

Exercise for Week #6: Contemplate & Act

Continue to meditate 15-20 minutes per day, with your choice on what type of meditation to conduct. Additionally, continue to practice self & other directed kindness and noting it each day to recognize your own ability to cultivate these humane values.

In addition, after contemplating one or multiple of the above questions, set a goal based on the second set of questions that would be an action towards living a life of presence, kindness, perpetual forgiveness, & love (see figure 10). One action you can choose to do each day is a Unification Imagery exercise, which is provided after figure 10.

Figure 10. Contemplation on Unification Log

Date	Item #	What action can you practice that would cultivate this?	What BETs got in the way? How could you respond in the future?
9/4/24	#2	I am attempting to live a healthier life, so I will allow myself one dessert per day instead of multiple	The positive BET of *"earned this"* came up. I acknowledged that it was a passing thought and let it go. I slipped up and ate more then I should. I forgave myself and contemplated what BET led to this.

Steps to Unification Imagery

Apply these steps after a few minutes of deep breathing to get yourself focused, calm, and alert. Don't forget in all of these trainings to do them with an attitude of kindness and acceptance of *"the way it is"*.

1. Slowly begin to visualize a painting with various swirling colors and strokes.

2. Imagine the details of the painting. Begin to examine each individual detail as best you can. What color, stroke type, and depth is it? Does it create a specific image for you?

3. If possible, even imagine the continuous flow of the painting as it is actively painted with each brush stroke.

4. As you begin to visualize each stroke, attempt to see how when they are first presented it is difficult to see how they are connected to the imagery, left, right, above, and below it.

5. With each inhale, allow your mind's eye to expand the imagery until you are able to see the larger painting.

6. Sooner or later you will be distracted and just return to the imagery

7. Visualize the details of each part of the painting. Maybe it is a visualization of a moment of your life, or even of you.

8. With each exhale allow yourself to see how each drop of paint, and stroke work together to create a singular image.

9. Return to your breath as needed to continue with the visualization.

10. As you begin to notice the entire image, recognize and forgive yourself for any flaw or error you find in the painting.

11. Allow each drop of paint and stroke to be as it is, and accept them individually, but more importantly, as one.

Creating Compassion

12. Observe how without taking in the entire painting / image, that the reality of the painting cannot be seen.

13. Thank yourself for the meditative experience at the end.

The goal of the above visualization is to see that all strokes of the painting are needed to create the unified image. Both the strokes we decided to create, and those that were created out of our control. Find forgiveness in the automatic strokes that we "feel" detract from the painting, but actually are just one singular element of the whole.

7. Compassion beyond Empathy

Compassion is many things, but immediate returns it is not

"Compassion is doing what is in the best interested of the whole connected individual, regardless of experiencing of natural suffering"

Mirror 7 - Compassion is Selfless, Even Towards One's Self

The term compassion and empathy are often used as synonyms; however, compassion is much more than empathy itself. Compassion is the driving positive energy towards understanding, being, and doing what is in the best interest of a being, regardless of experiencing of natural necessary suffering in the moment. Some of the qualities that encompass compassion are:

1. Empathy: the ability to emotionally feel and /or cognitively understand how a being is feeling, with the desire to reduce the suffering.

2. Forgiveness: the voluntary ability to accept an action, moment, or moments of time to allow you to move on and no longer be led by anger or resentment.

3. Patience: the virtue of taking one's time to allow BETs to naturally dissolve, without trying to force them.

4. Distress tolerance: the ability to hold and let go of a being's negative BETs instead of avoiding them through rejection, over indulgence, or ignoring.

5. Kindness: A series of actions, both verbal and non-verbal, that demonstrate that one is actively with a being during a moment of suffering (e.g., active listening, head nodding, hand touching, & etc.).

6. <u>Mindfulness</u>: the action of being completely present during a moment of suffering instead of jumping to "problem solving mode," unless the being wants to enter that mode.

As stated above, the being can be yourself and, in fact, should start with yourself as you are wherever you go.

The issue with cultivating compassion is we often attempt to do so during intense moments of distress. Of course many of us can do this for brief moments at a time, especially for those we deeply care about. However, when it comes to small moments of suffering, chronic suffering, and suffering of ourselves or those we do not care for, then this muscle is just not strong enough to bear it without dipping into the avoidance cycle during the events that trigger suffering or shortly after. For example:

1. After the loss of a loved one we can find ourselves being attentive to those around us that need it.

2. We can be empathetic, patient, tolerant of their distress, and kind.

3. This can be through action or non-action of just being there with them while they greave.

4. However, at the same time we may not be activating the compassionate self and giving ourselves the same qualities we are extending to others.

5. This can lead to a cycle of avoidance, leaving one vulnerable to extended suffering from the natural grief of losing a loved one.
    a. Over indulging in sensory pleasures, drugs, alcohol, or food.
    b. Rejecting negatives through suppression that may lead to it "bubbling up" when one least expects it.
    c. Ignoring the momentary moments of neutrality, that if not experienced deprive you of what other things you can do that may be helpful or harmful.

Thus, it is of the utmost importance to cultivate self-compassion and build that muscle by practicing its various components with the minor moments of suffering we experience each day. Spend some time with those neutral experiences of boredom to find out what may be helpful or harmful within them to be even more compassionate. For example, if you practice compassion on these small pains, especially those you would normally ignore, then you will develop an automatic habit of distress tolerance. By doing this over and over, all pain will get better because you will not automatically be adding suffering.

Daily Compassion Focused Exercises

Each component of compassion can be practiced in our daily experiences of suffering. Below are examples of how moments of suffering can be dissolved via activating the compassionate self (note: NAIL A BET may be used to become more aware of the cycle, with the above techniques used if it can be let go of). Think of the moments of suffering as a crying baby that you want to attend to versus an enemy you want to attack.

This baby is an apt metaphor for the young child within all of us that we need to recover and cultivate its property of the "first time mind" that is free of feelings like shame and doubt because each moment is experienced without selfish judgements, *"as new first time "* experience, thus seeing things *"the way it is"* free of being contaminated with distortions that result in adding suffering.

Below are some examples of how to utilize each component of compassion with a specific example.

- Failing to get a task done at home / work, which can lead to self-anger / shame, as well as anxiety that you aren't *"living up"* to what you *"should be."*

    o **Empathic** urge: deeply understand that you are fearing what this means about you and connecting this "failure" to your identity (note: see NAIL A BET to de-identify if possible).

    o **Forgive** yourself for being imperfect, as this action is not you and is just a temporary moment. There will be future moments to succeed, but both your failures and successes are not yours alone. Forgive yourself. This too will pass.

    o **Patience:** Be patient that you will have additional negative self-talk and find healthy ways to cope with it if you cannot de-identify from it.

    o **Distress Tolerance**: tolerate your negative emotions and do not avoid what will help you dissolve the natural emotion. If you need to talk with others about the "failure," talk with them. Others can often put our moments of distress into context (a.k.a. the reality as it is).

    o Be **kind** and find ways to let the emotion out naturally.

    o Remain **Mindful** with yourself and engage in frequent emotional check ins and repeat the above steps.
        - Use NAIL A BET as needed.
        - Use a self-compassion break or perfect nurturer (page 74) to help you dissolve the emotions.

"The most benefits occur through mindful practice of the Highest Humane Values of kindness, sharing, acceptance, & compassion for they activate our helping, healing, stabilizing powers."

Exercise for Week #7: Compassionate Self

The *"darkness within"* can be seen as hatred, anger, and shame directed towards ourselves, that often doesn't end at just emotional distress but many negative outcomes (e.g., severe drug / alcohol use, violence, and premature death). As such, we need to practice this daily so that when more significant stressors come up we will be prepared. At this point we have accumulated several strategies to do this, including:

1. Meditate 15-20 minutes per day. Utilize any one of the meditative practices provided in this or other texts.

2. Engage in one mindful activity per day that is not meditation. This can be reading, exercise, walking, listening to music, or just observing the world around you (e.g., observe the scenery as you are on a walk, without judgment)

3. Engage in emotional check-ins several times to day to be present with your emotional experiences.

4. Use NAIL A BET to let go of emotional experiences you can, so you continue accepting reality *"as it is."*

5. Engage in daily self and other directed kindness. Be aware of acts of kindness and find appreciation for them, no matter how small.

6. Practice contemplative meditation either through exchanges with others or within yourself on the deeper components of compassion and connectivity.

7. Engage in self & other directed compassion to dissolve negative emotions that you cannot let go of.
    a. Record the moment via NAIL A BET log (figure 5).
    b. Dissolve them through the components of compassion or a compassion based exercise / action (e.g., a moment of self-kindness versus self-hate).

Figure 5. NAIL A BET LOG

Notice-Non-Judgmentally	Accept as it is	Investigate or De-Identify	Learn & Let Go

Steps to Perfect Nurturer Imagery (Lee, 2005)

Similar to the deep breathing exercise, individuals who have strong visualization may benefit from using guided or self-guided imagery. Below are basic instructions on how to attempt guided imagery based on the same principles. Apply these steps after a few minutes of deep breathing.

1. Now what I would like you to do is begin to visualize a place that is perfectly safe for you. This can be a real place or a place that is completely of your own imagination.

2. It may be a place you've been to in your past such as a river, the beach, a cabin, or even your grandparents' home. Or it can be a place that you've only seen on TV or the movies or is of your own creation.

3. This is a place only for you and just brings you warmth and a sense of peace.

4. Begin to imagine items around you. If you're along a river maybe you notice how the river is flowing and the trees around you, maybe you notice small animals running past, or even the sound of the wind.

5. If you're in a cabin, maybe you notice the roaring fire in front of you and the warmth radiating as you lay, and just enjoy the gentle presence of the room.

6. Whatever your peaceful space is, make it your own. Utilizing each one of your senses to magnify this space. If it is a home you grew up in, or your grandparents' home, or a cabin, maybe you smell fire burning or food cooking. You can hear the crackling of a fire or the sounds of gentle music playing.

7. Imagine that you feel perfectly comfortable in this space, sitting or lying just in a position that feels comfortable for you.

8. At any time that you're getting pulled away from this visualization, just return to the sensation of your breath, as you breathe in and out.

9. With the next exhale just gently let go of the distraction and return to your visualization of this perfectly kind and warm space.

10. Now imagine that you know someone, a real or an imaginary individual, is coming to visit you.

11. This person could be someone who has passed or who is still living, a pet or grandparent, or a religious figure / deity that you find a connection with.

12. Specifically imagine someone who embodies all the elements of compassion is coming to visit you. Someone, who in this moment, only exists to be there for you.

13. If you're in a cabin or in a building, imagine that you can even see them out the window and you can see a smile across their face.

14. Become aware of your bodily reaction to this experience as they're approaching the room either through a window or down the way.

15. Maybe it's a fluttering of the heart, sweating of the palms, warming of the hands or face, or even just a gentle smile.

16. Just notice that experience and allow it to be.

17. Allow them to come into your space and greet them whatever way you feel you need to right now.

18. Imagine as best you can the expression of their face and the energy they give off.

19. Imagine that they sit next to you exactly at the distance you would like. If you would like them to embrace your hand, your arm, allow them to if that is right for you.

20. If they are smaller than you, or a pet, and you want to embrace them, then embrace them. Allow whatever is right for you.

21. Begin to imagine them speaking to you to give you the compassion that you need. Imagine that they begin to extend to you whatever elements of compassion you need right now.

    a. Imagine they are providing you the perseverance or strength you need.
    b. Allow them to say or extend the warmth and kindness you need in this moment.
    c. Let them provide patience and wisdom in the suffering you are experiencing in the here and now.
    d. Whatever additional element of compassion you need them to embody, allow them to do so and extend it to you.

22. Imagine that their entire presence is meant to be there just for you.

23. Begin to become aware of the emotional experience you are having as they extend these elements of compassion towards you.

24. Become aware of the physical sensations in your body that you feel when they do this. Maybe it is a fluttering of the heart, warming of the face or hands, or positive tension in your arms, almost as if you want to hug or reach out to them.

25. Whatever the sensation is, allow it come, be, and go.

26. Now imagine that they approach slightly closer to tell you what you need to hear right now.

27. If you have difficulty hearing anything that is okay as well. Just enjoy their company.

28. If they did say something imagine that they whispered it to you and that you can hold onto it whenever you need it.

29. Allow yourself to sit with this being as long as you need.

30. Eventually they will depart, but know they are always able to come to you when you need their strength.

31. Allow them to gently depart as you begin to focus on your breath again.

32. Breathing in, and out.

33. If you feel comfortable doing so, place your hand over your heart and silently repeat whatever phrase of compassion they extended to you.

34. Slowly allow the imagery to dissolve as you return to the room.

35. Taking one last deep breath in, and out.

Practice the above compassion exercises daily to cultivate a daily practice of self and other kindness so that you will be prepared when more difficult stressors face you. Feel free to return to the pervious chapters as needed as well. Remember, self-growth will be rewarded, but only in its own time, so be patient with the practice and continue to accept reality as it is to live a happy, healthy, and compassionate life.

About the Authors

Cyril M J Puhalla MD, is recently retired with a previous practices in Dunmore-Scranton, PA. & clinical instructor of medical students attending The Geisinger Commonwealth Medical School in Scranton Pa. He was born and raised in the same city where he practiced child, adolescent & adult psychiatry. He is a Board-Certified Child Adolescent & Adult Psychiatrist with over 50 years of experience. He is a graduate of the University of Scranton & Jefferson Medical School, in Philadelphia Pa. and completed post graduated training there in child, adolescent and adult psychiatry. He has been classically psychoanalyzed & had training at the Philadelphia Psychoanalytic Association. He is also trained in individual, group, family, cognitive-behavior, and hypnotherapy & is accomplished in creative clinical psychopharmacology especially in children and adolescents.

Alexander A. Puhalla, Ph.D., son of Dr. Cyril Puhalla, is a licensed clinical psychologist who has nearly a decade of experience with mindfulness based cognitive psychotherapy across psychiatric diagnosis. Additionally, he has created and implemented mindfulness and compassion-based groups for those with various psychological conditions, including, but not limited to, those with posttraumatic stress disorder, substance use disorders, anxiety disorders and mood disorders. He has implemented these groups across levels of care (e.g., inpatient unit, residential care, intensive outpatient, and general outpatient) and has utilized them within individual work as well. Beyond Dr. Puhalla's clinical expertise, he has over a dozen publications across aggression, self-aggression, posttraumatic stress disorder, and negative self-evaluative emotions. Dr. Puhalla works at The Veterans Affairs and actively trying to integrate compassion focused interventions across levels of care for veterans with concurrent trauma and substance use disorder symptoms.

Resources and Recommended Readings

1. Allen,R.C."Emily-Dickinson-Accidental-Buddhist"-Victoria,Canada:Trafford Pub 2007.
2. Brach, Tara. "Radical Acceptance." New York: Bantam Books, 2003
3. Gunaratana, B H. "Eight Mindful Steps to Happiness." Boston: Wisdom Pub, 2001
4. Hagen, Steve. "Buddhism Plain & Simple." Boston: Charles Tuttle, 1997.
5. Gyatso, G K. "Meditation Handbook" Glen Spey, NY: Tharpa Publications, 2001
6. Hairfield,-Steven-"The-12-Sacred-Principles-of-Karma"-Selah,WA:-Innercircle -2009
7. Kyabgon,Traleg-"Karma-What it is, What it is, what It Isn't"-Shambahala, Co-2015
8. Lama, Dali. "Becoming Enlightened". New York: Atria Books, 2009
9. Loy, David. "Lack & Transcendence." Amherst, NY: Humanity Books. 1996
10. Merton, Thomas. "New Seeds of Contemplation" NY: New Directions, 2007
11. Moffitt, Phillip. "Dancing with Life" Rodale Press,2008
12. Puhalla, C.M, & Puhalla, A.A. "Life is Painful, Make Suffering Optional!: Answering Life's Critical Questions with Principles for Health Happiness & Peace of Mind & Mindfulness Practice." Independently Published, 2023
13. Sumedho,Ajahn-"The Four Nobel Truths",Amaravanti,1999
14. Sumedho,Ajahn-"The Mind & The Way" Wisdom Pub. Mass,1995
15. Sumedho,Ajahn"The Way it Is", Amaravanti, 1991
16. Rosenberg, L. "Breath-by-Breath."Boston:Shambala.1998
17. Suzuki, S. "Zen Mind, Beginner's Mind." Boston: Shambala Publishing. 2011
18. Tsering, G T. "Buddhist Psychology." Boston: Wisdom Publication. 2006.
19. Williams-Teasdale-Kabat-Zinn"Mindful-Way-though-Depression-NY-Guilford-Press-2010

References

Au, T. M., Sauer-Zavala, S., King, M. W., Petrocchi, N., Barlow, D. H., & Litz, B. T. (2017). Compassion-based therapy for trauma-related shame and posttraumatic stress: Initial evaluation using a multiple baseline design. *Behavior therapy*, *48*(2), 207-221.

Gilbert, P. (2009). Introducing compassion-focused therapy. *Advances in psychiatric treatment*, *15*(3),199-208.

Gunaratana, H. (2017). *Loving-kindness in plain English: The practice of Metta*. Simon and Schuster.

Gyatso, G. K. (2019). *The Mirror of Dharma with Additions: How to find the real meaning of human life*. Tharpa Publications US.

Hochswender, W., Martin, G., & Morino, T. (2001). *The Buddha in your mirror: Practical Buddhism and the search for self*. Middleway Press.

Lee, D. A. (2005). The perfect nurturer: A model to develop a compassionate mind within the context of cognitive therapy. In *Compassion* (pp. 326-351). Routledge.

Millard, L. A., Wan, M. W., Smith, D. M., & Wittkowski, A. (2023). The effectiveness of compassion focused therapy with clinical populations: A systematic review and meta-analysis. *Journal of Affective Disorders*, *326*, 168-192.

Appendix

All handouts are provided here for your ease. It may be helpful to separate them from the book or create a copy for you to bring around with you.

Figure 1. The 12 Basic Laws
The Laws represent "the way it is," though 12 separate principles that are interconnected.

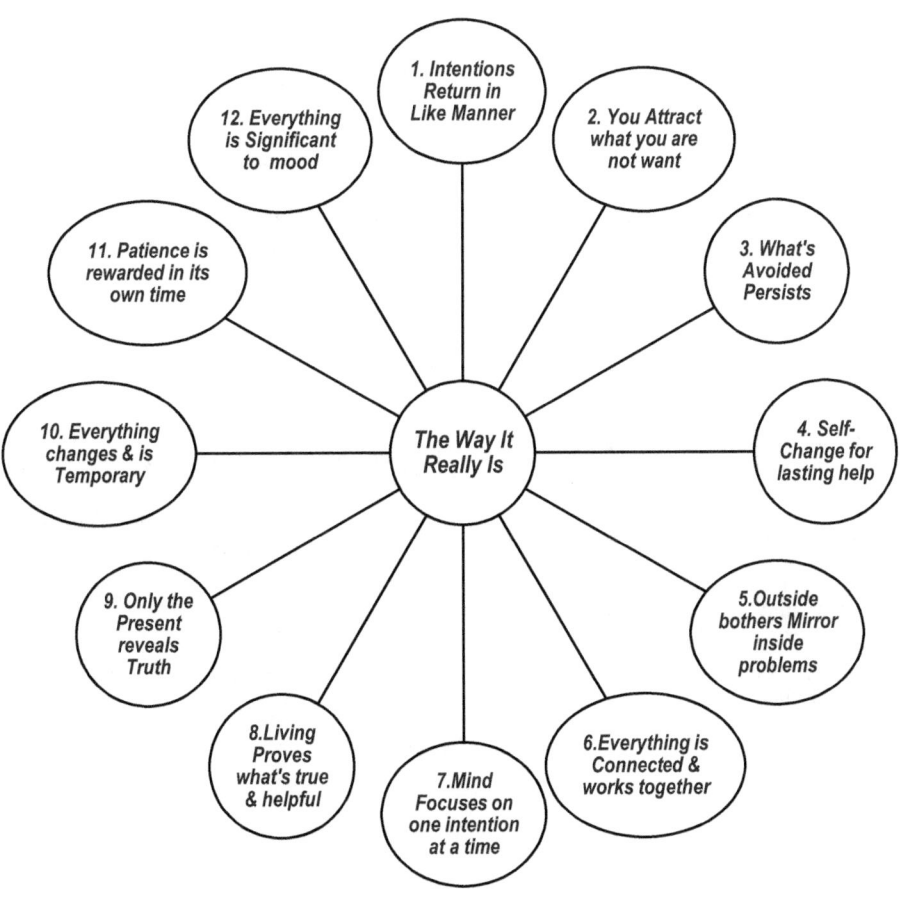

Figure 2. Removing harm of Cyclic Self-Destructiveness by Letting Go of Attachments of Separate Self with Compassion

Cycle of Self-Destructiveness: Separate Self	Steps for Health, Happiness, & Peace: Connected Self
☐ Unaware that avoiding painful feelings of *"the way it is"* is harmful	☐ Mindful awareness of harm of avoidance
☐ Pain is not *"what I want"*	☐ Pains accepted mindfully with compassion
☐ Only perceive what I want as the pleasures & avoid pains	☐ *"the way it really is"* there is no pleasure without pain, no pain without pleasure
☐ Separate oneself from pains	☐ Stay connected to pain & pleasure
☐ Desire makes new pleasure exist & pain not exist over humane values	☐ Humane intentions towards kindness, sharing, and connection
☐ Become trapped in thinking mode to avoid the reality as it is.	☐ Shift from thinking to mindful dissolving & compassion
☐ New feelings personalized as friend or foe	☐ Feelings as impersonal energy
☐ Attach to new feelings to ignore neutrals	☐ Let feelings fully come
☐ Over indulge in positves & reject negatives	☐ Let feelings be as they are
☐ Seperate self becomes more powerful	☐ Compassion feeling of painful energy to let the attachment go!
☐ Life's solutions contaminated with uncertainty, fear, depression, addiction & anger	☐ No extra uncertainty, fear, depression, addictivness, & anger
☐ Self is unaware of harmful avoidance which fuels a new cycle	☐ No Cycle - instead Health, Happiness, & Peace Of Mind

Figure 3. Emotion Log (NAIL made simple):

Date	**N**otice & Allow (Emotion)	**I**nvestigate (Thoughts / Urges)	**L**earn (Usual reaction vs. Alternatives)
8/10/24	Anxiety Fear	I am going to fail this test no matter what. Avoid studying	Usually I will focus on my anxiety or do something else. I could just sit and study for a bit.

Figure 4. Mindfulness Practice Log

Date	Meditation Practice	Mindful Living Practice	Notes (how did engaging in presence feel or effect you?)
8/17/24	3x today for 5 minutes. 1x at bedtime.	While swimming I only paid attention to my body's experience	1. It helped me fall alseep. 2. When I did it before my meeting I was calmer. 3. I enjoyed my breakfast more.

Figure 5. NAIL A BET LOG

Notice-Non-Judgmentally	Accept as it is	Investigate or De-Identify	Learn & Let Go
Feeling depressed	It is just a moment of sadness	I miss loved ones, but this is just a momentary thought not who I permanently am	This will pass, just like all emotions. Focus on what I have control over.

Figure 6. Meditation Log

Date	Meditation Type	What BETs distracted you the most?	How can you instill greater compassion next practice?

Figure 7. The Separate Self vs. The Connected Self

Seperate Self	Connected Self
☐ *"way you want it to be"*	☐ *"the way it really is,"*
☐ Motivated by desire	☐ Humane motivations
☐ Desire is never Satisfied	☐ Humaneness is satisfaction
☐ Avoidance causes distress	☐ Acceptance as stress relief
☐ Hold on to pleasure	☐ Satisfaction is letting go
☐ Satisfaction is outside	☐ Satisfaction in the Mind
☐ Avoid pain to harm	☐ Take in Pain to Help
☐ Judgemental biased	☐ Accepts all equally
☐ Progressive anger	☐ Kind patient peaceful
☐ Un-caring to suffering	☐ Altruistic compassion
☐ Illness Ageing Death	☐ Health Happiness Peace
☐ Avoid to Cycle Suffering	☐ Acceptance ends suffering

Figure 8. Loving-Kindness Meditation & Action Log

Date	Meditation Type	Loving-Kindness Action	What Judgements or BETs came up?

Figure 9. Loving-Kindness Meditation & Action Log

Date	Meditation Type	Loving-Kindness Action (Towards self? Shared with others?)	What Judgements got in the way? Were you able to forgive & let go?

Figure 10. Contemplation on Unification Log

Date	Item #	What action can you practice that would cultivate this?	What BETs got in the way? How could you respond in the future?
9/4/24	#2	I am attempting to live a healthier life, so I will allow myself one dessert per day instead of multiple	The positive BET of *"earned this"* came up. I acknowledged that it was a passing thought and let it go. I slipped up and ate more then I should. I forgave myself and contemplated what BET led to this.

www.ingramcontent.com/pod-product-compliance
Lightning Source LLC
Chambersburg PA
CBHW050325230526
45471CB00005B/2351